Dyslexic AND UN-Stoppable
The Cookbook

Dyslexic
AND
UN-Stoppable
The Cookbook

Revealing Our Secrets—How Having
Healthier Brains and Lifestyles
Helps US Overcome Dyslexia

Lucie M. Curtiss, R.N.
Douglas C. Curtiss, M.D., FAAP

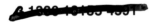

(M·J)
New York

Dyslexic AND UN-Stoppable The Cookbook
Revealing Our Secrets—How Having Healthier Brains and Lifestyles Helps US Overcome Dyslexia

Published in New York, New York, by Morgan James Publishing. Morgan James and The Entrepreneurial Publisher are trademarks of Morgan James, LLC.
www.MorganJamesPublishing.com

The Morgan James Speakers Group can bring authors to your live event. For more information or to book an event visit The Morgan James Speakers Group at www.TheMorganJamesSpeakersGroup.com.

To take advantage of all of the extras, including supplemental videos, visit:
www.DyslexicAndUnstoppable.com
Click on: Book Extras
Enter the password: Unstoppable2

Children, REMEMBER: You *always* need adult supervision in the kitchen while cooking and baking! Always.

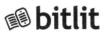

A **free** eBook edition is available
with the purchase of this print book.

CLEARLY PRINT YOUR NAME ABOVE IN UPPER CASE
Instructions to claim your free eBook edition:
1. Download the BitLit app for Android or iOS
2. Write your name in **UPPER CASE** on the line
3. Use the BitLit app to submit a photo
4. Download your eBook to any device

ISBN 978-1-63047-559-8 paperback
ISBN 978-1-63047-609-0 eBook
Library of Congress Control Number:
2015905162

Cover Design by:
Rachel Lopez
www.r2cdesign.com

Interior Design by:
Bonnie Bushman
bonnie@caboodlegraphics.com

In an effort to support local communities and raise awareness and funds, Morgan James Publishing donates a percentage of all book sales for the life of each book to Habitat for Humanity Peninsula and Greater Williamsburg

Get involved today, visit
www.MorganJamesBuilds.com

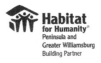

Habitat for Humanity®
Peninsula and
Greater Williamsburg
Building Partner

This book is dedicated to the parents of dyslexic children. Your patience, courage, perseverance, resilience, and determination are the keys to bringing hope by helping kids overcome dyslexia. Your willingness to investigate and research solutions to help your child achieve his or her highest potential is the greatest gift you can give as a parent.

Thank you for joining our community and allowing us to be part of your journey.

We are forever grateful for your commitment to your child's success in life!

Contents

Foreword

For the longest time I have been dreaming about publishing a novel. The plot has been seared in my head for as long as I can remember, probably from the time I was in college, learning math and biology and classic Greek. While I was still practicing medicine, I developed the habit of accumulating notes on scraps of paper. Tons of them. But I never found the time or was too tired to sit down and start turning them into a book. Since I retired some years ago, every chance I get, I spend a couple of hours trying to put my ideas on paper. At first I thought after a year or so I would be done. A hundred and fifty pages—two hundred at the most—that would almost write themselves. Dream on. After all those years I am still spending several hours almost every day on the darn project. One of the problems I have is that I probably delete more than I keep. Nevertheless the book already contains more than double the number of pages I was planning on writing and I am not even sure I have reached the middle of it yet.

So when my daughter Lucie told me not so long ago that she was writing a book, I thought, *Yeah, sure! Lucie, who had such a hard time reading! Writing a book? While at the same time raising a family and managing her husband's practice?* But a few months later, with a smile on her face, she handed me a copy of *Dyslexic AND UN-Stoppable*, confirming to me—once more—that she really is unstoppable.

As I was still in the process of getting used to the idea, she recently announced that she was about to publish a second book, this time co-authored by her own daughter Chloé. The thought that went through my mind this time was a quote from Gomer Pile: *Gaw-ol-ly!* How can that be? Even my granddaughter is getting published before me! This has to be part of a conspiracy.

Seriously, when I read *Dyslexic AND UN-Stoppable*, Lucie's first book, my first reaction was: finally, somebody is doing something to raise awareness about dyslexia. I remembered going to parent/teachers meetings and complaining to her teachers and at least once even to the school principal about her confusing certain letters, mostly c's and s's, or writing numbers backward. The replies I would get were always similar: "She needs to pay more attention," or "Don't worry. She'll grow out of it." Or some other excuse. Not being an expert in the field of education, I didn't dare insist that maybe something else could possibly be done about this.

I am sure thousands, if not millions, of bright kids have been treated as stupid or lazy or have been bullied or even dropped out of school because nobody knew or would take a moment to try to detect what was happening to them.

Luckily times have changed. And now numerous well-educated people have devised methods and means of identifying the condition and even making use of it as a tool to find new and better solutions to the problems of this world.

Possibly the most valuable role *Dyslexic AND UN-Stoppable* will play is that it will help parents and teachers recognize early kids who are—or may be—affected with this disorder. Early detection and consultation with experts (before irreparable damage is done) will then help them live lives as interesting and fulfilling as anybody else.

I see Lucie's cookbook as another worthwhile tool in the arsenal to combat prejudice against dyslexia and other learning disorders, and to help the kids affected overcome this inconvenience.

The cookbook is interesting and easy to read. It contains recipes for nutritious, easy to prepare, fun to eat, and delicious snacks and even meals. My favorite is undeniably number eight: *Crêpes à la Maman* (drowning in Canadian maple syrup). If unavailable, American maple syrup may be used as a somewhat acceptable substitute. (Obviously this is just my attempt at a little Canadian humor.)

To make the most wholesome choices, the authors suggest using only organic ingredients and to avoid those with additives such as artificial coloring, preservatives, and especially drugs like hormones, antibiotics, and others. Also, they recommend avoiding foods containing GMOs. But if you've at least looked for organic food in the grocery store, you know that it's expensive.

Don't let this discourage you from reading this book or using the recipes. Buy the best ingredients you can afford and just add the secret ingredient[1] the authors neglected to mention. Use lots of it. (I'm sure they use plenty themselves.)

As an added bonus, the book contains names and pictures of a number of famous people thought to have been dyslexic, with some of their memorable quotes.

Finally I urge you to read the epilogue. It contains excellent advice on how to detect dyslexia early in your child and, if he or she is affected, to help him or her overcome the inconvenience associated with it.

All in all, a lot of useful and pleasant reading. Enjoy!

Médard Bérubé, MD, LMCC, DPH

P'pa and Granp'pa

---

1   Even myself, I didn't dare mention the name of the ingredient because it's a four-letter word. A hint to help you guess what it is: it starts with the letter L and it rhymes with dove.

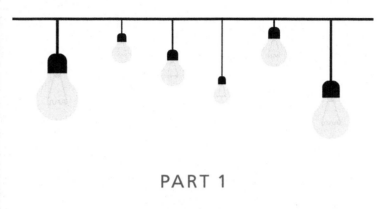

PART 1

Our Mission

CHAPTER 1

Who Are We?

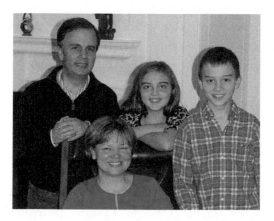

Lucie M. Curtiss

My name is Lucie Curtiss, and I'm dyslexic. I've been coping with dyslexia for over forty years. Despite my struggles in school when I was young, I managed to become successful in my life. I finally realized I was dyslexic when I was in my mid-twenties. With fierce determination and a desire to succeed no matter what, I was able to overcome dyslexia and accomplish my dreams.

Also, my husband and I discovered that our son Félix-Alexander (FéZander) was dyslexic. So for the past twelve years, we've been helping him succeed, and the results are showing up in every aspect of his life. It's wonderful to see him blossom. Now we want to share our journey with other dyslexics and hope what we've learned may help someone else succeed.

> You can learn more about Lucie's personal journey with dyslexia by reading her full story ("The Author's Journey with Dyslexia") in our first book, *Dyslexic AND UN-Stoppable: How Dyslexia Helps Us Create the Life of Our Dreams and How YOU Can Do It Too!*

Dr. Douglas C. Curtiss

I am Dr. Douglas Curtiss, an Ivy League–trained pediatrician who learned traditional Western medicine. As a student of personal development, I began to look at complementary medicine techniques to incorporate into my practice. When our son was discovered to be dyslexic, I worked with my wife, Lucie, to find the best methods, both traditional and complementary, to help our son overcome dyslexia and become an excellent student, moving to the top of his class. In this book, Lucie has developed delicious recipes to help your dyslexic child. I show you the science behind these recommendations so that you can make educated choices to help your child rise to his or her fullest potential.

> You can learn more about Dr. Curtiss ("A Pediatrician's and Dad's Perspective") in our first book called *Dyslexic AND UN-Stoppable: How Dyslexia Helps Us Create the Life of Our Dreams and How YOU Can Do It Too!*

Félix-Alexander C. Curtiss

My name is Félix-Alexander. My friends call me Félix, and my family calls me Baba and FéZander. I do have many nicknames and I like them all.

After all the hard work, I now use dyslexia to my advantage. To keep me going, my mom and sister make healthy food. This food not only tastes great, it keeps my body healthy and me energized. This makes a win-win-win situation. As a dyslexic, I have endless ideas. My mom and sister cook great food to keep me energized, and I am able to complete my ideas.

I love taking care of my body and myself. Being healthy is important to me. I always check the ingredient lists on packages to make sure the food is healthy and doesn't have a bunch of chemicals. If the list contains five or less ingredients and I can read them, I know it's okay for me to eat.

Since this food tastes so good, there is no reason for me to eat fast food. I can't believe that such good food could taste so amazing. These recipes are the best in the world, as far as I'm concerned.

> You can learn more about Félix-Alexander's full story and journey with dyslexia in our first book, *Dyslexic AND UN-Stoppable: How Dyslexia Helps Us Create the Life of Our Dreams and How YOU Can Do It Too!*

Chloé K. Curtiss ("Cookie")

I'm Chloé and I'm ten years old. I'm Félix's little sister. The two of us are best friends and always help each other out. When I was born and Félix was a little boy, he nicknamed me "Cookie" because he couldn't say "Chloé." Now my whole family calls me Cookie, even my cousins.

I like that my mom and dad let me help out with the drawing and cooking. I designed Sparky the Owl and the rainbow picture on the first book.

I love to cook with my mom, and making the videos for this book was a lot of fun. I made most of the recipes with the help of my mom, and my brother loved to eat all of the food we made, especially the peanut butter cookies!

CHAPTER 2

Where Does Dyslexic AND UN-Stoppable Come From?

Dyslexic AND UN-Stoppable, LLC, was born out of our desire to see dyslexic children like our son overcome dyslexia. We've done the research, took the classes, and learned the tools. Now we want to pass this great information to other dyslexics and their families so they also can succeed and become UN-Stoppable.

Learning where to get the services and how to help our son was a long process of trial and error. So we figured it would be nice to help other parents and teachers find the information they needed in the fastest time possible. The sooner parents can identify dyslexia in their child, the greater the chance of success in overcoming it.

We hope that by sharing our journey with the world, we will be able to help other dyslexic children. We realize that some children are more severely challenged than our son, but if we can at least bring them hope, help them find their passion, help them find their unique gifts, or help save their self-esteem, then we will have served our purpose. We just need to open one little door for the possibilities to show up. We want to remind **dyslexics** that they are **SMART** and can do anything they put their minds to!

We have one main mission at Dyslexic AND UN-Stoppable: to help dyslexics rediscover their inner power and become UN-Stoppable.

The *Dyslexic AND UN-Stoppable* book series is designed to provide dyslexics with all the information, tools, and strategies we learned along this journey to help them overcome dyslexia. Living with dyslexia is a lifelong journey. We can overcome some of the challenges, but dyslexia will always remain part of us. For this reason, we will keep gathering the information, and we will continue sharing it with you. This is just the beginning for Dyslexic AND UN-Stoppable. Stay connected with us to remain updated about our new resources, such as Dr. Curtiss's empowering book for his dyslexic patients, which will be out soon.

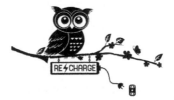

Sparky the Owl: Company Mascot

Our mission at Dyslexic AND UN-Stoppable is to help dyslexic children rediscover their inner power and become UN-Stoppable.

CHAPTER 3

Why We Wrote
This Second Book

Our first book, *Dyslexic AND UN-Stoppable: How Dyslexia Helps Us Create the Life of Our Dreams and How YOU Can Do It Too!*, gave parents and teachers concrete examples of tools and strategies that helped our son overcome difficulties with writing, reading, math, and speech, and to help parents get the services they need for their children to succeed in the public schools.

Our goal for this second book in the *Dyslexic AND UN-Stoppable series* is to complement the first book. Overcoming dyslexia is a continual journey, so we recommend reading our first book in conjunction with this book to get maximum benefits and results.

In this book, we will focus mainly on nutritional facts, healthy recipes, and how to identify the healthy ingredients that are beneficial for improving your odds of overcoming dyslexia, as well as the non-healthy ingredients to avoid. We've adapted recipes we like to eat to provide our son who is dyslexic with the best nutrients to keep his brain functioning at its best. These recipes are designed for the whole family to enjoy. Like most people, we are a busy, on-the-go family, and time is of the essence. We need to make meals that we all enjoy and benefit from, because in the end, we all need and want a healthy brain, dyslexic or otherwise.

After years of research, we now realize that using as many pure and simple ingredients as possible is the key to getting maximum benefit from our foods.

We can only speak from our own experience, but we've noticed that by removing as many of certain ingredients from FéZander's diet as possible, he has made great improvements in his ability to concentrate and focus.

On a side note: I (Lucie/Mom) also noticed an improvement in my health as an adult living with dyslexia when I changed my eating habits. The better I eat, the better I cope with life and work-related stresses, which in return means I'm better able to concentrate and deal with problems as they arise.

When possible, we eat foods that contain no artificial dyes, no preservatives, no chemicals, no added salt, no aluminum, no antibiotics, and no growth hormones, and that are not genetically modified (non-GMO).

Some examples of foods we like to use are organic foods, wild caught fish, free-range eggs, and raw veggies and fruits. Basically we use foods in their purest and simplest form to preserve their nutrients.

As we said above, we can only speak from our own experience. Of course, we wouldn't expect that what we are doing to help our son will automatically help all other children overcome dyslexia. We are all unique individuals with different degrees of difficulties, but our hope is that we can help even a little.

One of our mentors always starts his courses and camps by stating something like, "Don't believe a word I say; this is my experience only. This is what works for me, and it doesn't mean it will work for you." When we first heard him say that, we thought, *What? What does that mean? What is he trying to tell us?* Today, we get it. Our mentor wants to help as many people as he can, but he also realizes that it's simply impossible to help everyone all the time. We are all at different places and on different paths in our lives. Some will benefit from our work and some won't, and we're okay with that. Some will hear similar information from someone else and understand it more clearly from them. In the end, as long as we do our best, that's all that matters.

The suggestions in this book are what work for us! We are not "recommending" anything. We are simply offering recipe ideas that have benefitted us. **Again, it's important that you do your own research!**

You always need to do your own research and make your own decisions about your food choices. We are all unique and different.

Since as dyslexics, we LOVE visuals, we decided to follow the successful trend of our first book by including video instructions on our website for each recipe.

For most recipes, "Cookie" (our daughter Chloé) will show you step-by-step how to make these delicious meals.

Visit our website www.DyslexicAndUnstoppable.com to view the videos for each recipe. Each video is titled with the same name as the recipe.

Recipe #1: Baba's "Almost Famous" Chocolate Torpedo Sandwich
Recipe #2: Tuna Melts My Way!
Recipe #3: Super-Easy Shrimp Stir-Fry
Recipe #4: Scrumptious Salmon
Recipe #5: An Old Favorite: Smoked Salmon Bagel
Recipe #6: Meat Tacos with "Dip-Dip"
Recipe #7: Fish Tacos with "Dip-Dip"
Recipe #8: *Crêpes à la Maman*
Recipe #9: Super-Easy Banana Bread
Recipe #10: Chloé's "Surprise" Peanut Butter Cookies

As a Bonus, this book also includes information on *nine* **Well-Known Dyslexics**[2] *who changed the world and made a huge impact.* After each recipe, you will find one of them profiled, along with their "claim to fame" and a few quotes from them!

Remember, being healthy is the key to conquering obstacles in life. The healthier we are, the better we are able to cope with and manage difficulties and become successful. The healthier we eat, the better we feel. The better we feel, the better we can face challenges and surmount them. And a healthy brain is a happy brain. Surely a happy and healthy brain helps to overcome dyslexia!

We hope that after reading this book you will also be able to come up with new simple and yummy recipe ideas your family will enjoy, and we hope you will share them with us on our website DyslexicAndUnstoppable.com. Let's all work together to overcome dyslexia!

---

2   Some of the Well-Known Dyslexics mentioned in this cookbook have confirmed their dyslexia in the media. Others may not have been clearly identified as having dyslexia. However, researchers have reviewed available evidence, and many have come to the conclusion that they did in fact have dyslexia. We leave it to you, the reader, to decide for yourself, as our main reason for including them is to inspire children with dyslexia.

How to Best Read and Utilize
This Book for Optimal Results

Visit DyslexicAndUnstoppable.com, and check out the video for each recipe.

Password: Unstoppable2

CHAPTER 4

What Do Healthy Foods and Diet Have to Do with Dyslexia, Anyway?

Most parents understand the importance of good nutrition for their children's school performance. Many parents even know what nutrients boost brain power and concentration. The big question is how to get these nutritious foods into their children. This is why we wrote this cookbook. We wanted you to have simple, easy-to-make recipes of delicious meals and snacks that your children will eat and that will help improve their performance at school and in life. In this chapter, I (Doug) hope to explain why we included various recipes and ingredients, what the individual nutrients do to help brain function, and what the research has shown. We will look at specific nutrients and what their effect has been shown to be on the brain. At the end of the chapter we will include some of the controversies surrounding certain ingredients so that you can make an informed decision for your child.

Before we delve into individual ingredients and their effect on brain function, I want to lay out some of the general principles of this book. First, whenever possible, we have used organic, natural ingredients with no preservatives and very little in the way of additives. Essentially we feel that the closer the ingredients are to what nature has made, the more nutritious they are. Therefore, whenever possible, we have tried to include whole grains, unrefined sugars, and foods that require no cooking. This helps maintain the food in its most nutritious state.

> You can learn more about how to help your child with dyslexia by reading the chapters ("A Pediatrician's and Dad's Perspective" and "Tools and Strategies") in our first book called *Dyslexic AND UN-Stoppable: How Dyslexia Helps Us Create the Life of Our Dreams and How YOU Can Do It Too!*

Basic Principles and Why They Are Important

1. **Whole grains:** The use of whole grains is important for general health for two reasons. First, the whole grain has all of the fiber, which helps improve the health of the colon. By improving colonic movement, the fiber in whole grains helps move waste through the bowel more regularly. The second benefit of whole grain products, as opposed to products manufactured with refined, white

flour, is that whole grains cause a slower rise in blood sugar, which then mutes the body's secretion of insulin. This should help your child avoid that "crash" in energy that some children experience mid-morning.

2. **Minimizing sugars and using unrefined sugars wherever possible:** Using less refined sugar may require some adjustment. However, with time your children will appreciate a variety of tastes in the food and will miss that sugary flavor less. Still, there are ways to sweeten foods without sugar. Using maple sugar or coconut sugar adds the sweetness, as well as a slightly more complex flavor, and these sugars do have some trace elements missing in white sugar.

3. **Organic ingredients:** While organic products may be more expensive, they have the benefit of fewer additives. They are also usually grown with fewer pesticides.

Foods to Avoid

1. **Artificial dyes:** There has been controversy over the health effects of artificial dyes in foods. However, with the rise in the diagnosis of attention problems in conjunction with the increase in the use of these dyes, there has been interest in whether these artificial dyes may play a role. Many studies have been too small to definitively tell if these chemicals affect attention. However, there was one double-blind, placebo-

controlled study, which is the best type of study to minimize bias. The study was performed in England and looked at preschoolers and elementary school children. The kids were randomized to drink either natural fruit juices or those with various artificial colors with and without the preservative sodium benzoate. The children who drank the juice with the artificial ingredients were found to have a mild but significant increase in hyperactivity during the six weeks they were observed. Given the amount of concentration that most children with dyslexia need for school, it only makes sense to avoid these chemicals.

2. **Artificial flavors.** There have been numerous studies showing the deleterious effects of artificial flavors on attention and concentration in children. A study by Egger et al in the journal *The Lancet* found that artificial flavors were the substances that most commonly exacerbated concentration problems in children.

Nutrients for Optimal Brain Health

So, which nutrients have been shown to be beneficial for brain health and memory? Have any nutrients specifically been shown to improve attention and dyslexia? As with everything in medicine, the science can be complex, contradictory, and confusing. Here we will lay out some basic facts, as well as our interpretation of the facts.

1. **Omega-3 fatty acids:** There are two omega-3 fatty acids: eicosapentanoic acid (EPA) and docosahexanoic acid (DHA). These fatty acids make up 20 percent of the weight of the brain. They have been shown to be beneficial for heart health (lowering blood pressure and triglycerides) and prenatal health (improving brain and eye development in fetuses). However, recent research has shown a benefit in children with ADHD, dyslexia, and dyspraxia. The Dyslexia Research Trust in England recently concluded a study. Their Oxford-Durham study (http://www.dyslexic.org.uk/research-nutrition.html) was a double-blind, randomized controlled trial (RCT). It showed an improvement in reading, spelling, and concentration in children with dyspraxia after three months of taking supplemental fish oil capsules. In addition, their reading grade level jumped by nine months over this three-month period.

What are some sources of omega-3 fatty acids?

- Fish, especially the so-called fatty fish like salmon and tuna
- Nuts
- Oils

- Beans
- Vegetables, especially broccoli, cauliflower, and winter squash
- Flaxseed, which actually contains a different fatty acid called alpha-linolenic acid (ALA). The ALA is partly broken down by the body to omega-3s.

2. **Vitamin E.** This fat-soluble vitamin has been shown in many studies to decrease the risk of dementia-related disorders, such as Alzheimer's disease. Since it has been shown to prevent the decline in brain function in older people, there has been interest in using it to improve focus and concentration in children. Studies have not yet been conclusive, and since vitamin E can be stored in the body's fat cells, you don't want to overdo it. However, eating healthy foods that are high in vitamin E may be helpful.

Great sources of vitamin E include:

- Shellfish
- Nuts, such as almonds
- Spinach
- Fish
- Avocados

3. **B vitamins:** The various B vitamins are vital to brain health. These vitamins are important in the formation of neurotransmitters that the brain cells use to communicate with each other. B vitamins include vitamin B6, vitamin B12, and folic acid.

Foods rich in the various B vitamins include:

- Beans and peas (folic acid, vitamin B6)
- Citrus juices (folic acid)
- Dark green leafy vegetables (folic acid, vitamin B6)
- Fish (vitamin B6, vitamin B12)

4. **Magnesium:** There have been studies showing a positive effect of magnesium supplementation on focus and concentration in children. A 1997 study by Starobrat-Hermelin et al showed an improvement in concentration in children given magnesium supplementation.

Excellent natural sources of magnesium include:

- Fish, such as halibut and mackerel
- Cocoa
- Nuts, such as almonds and cashews
- Seeds, such as pumpkin seeds

Some Controversies Surrounding Nutrition and Brain Health

There are some areas of controversy in nutrition, especially as it applies to brain health, attention, and dyslexia. Some of this controversy stems from conflicting results of various studies, and some from the misinterpretation of studies that have been performed. Wherever possible, we have tried to clear up the confusion. If definitive answers are not available, we will give you what evidence there is so that you can come to an informed decision yourself.

Omega-6 versus Omega-3 Fatty Acids

Both omega-6 and omega-3 fatty acids are considered essential fatty acids since our bodies cannot make these fatty acids. Therefore it is necessary for us to eat foods that contain them so that we can maintain proper nutrition. The key, however, is to maintain a proper balance of these two varieties of fatty acids. Since the average American diet is already high in omega-6 fatty acids, we have focused on ways of increasing the omega-3s to obtain the proper ratio.

Flaxseed

As soon as any food is studied for its nutritional benefit, there are people who come out against it. Flaxseed and flaxseed oil are examples of this. Here are some reasons people have come out against flaxseed:

- It has phytoestrogens that people worry can be harmful, especially in women at risk for breast cancer.
- It contains the fatty acid ALA, which is only partially converted to DHA and EPA.
- There is concern that flaxseed oil is easily oxidized if heated.

We use flaxseed oil in conjunction with fish oils and olive oils, and feel we have reached a good balance in our lives. In addition, when we add flaxseed oil, we do not cook it to avoid oxidizing it.

In the end, parents need to weigh the available facts and come to their own conclusion about what is best for their children. Our goal in this cookbook is to provide you with tasty recipes that promote excellent nutrition, which we have found have improved focus and concentration in our son with dyslexia. Most importantly, these recipes take into consideration the lives of busy parents and their kids. We have perfected these recipes to be easy to prepare, using the best ingredients in an economical way. Thus, busy working parents can easily make these dishes and still watch their bottom line. Also, we have tried the recipes out on our son, who started out with very finicky tastes. We have found that he loves these dishes and with time has begun to expand his repertoire. Give them a try, and then visit us at www.DyslexicAndUnstoppable.com and let us know what you think.

You can learn more about food, nutrition, and helpful supplements by reading the chapter "Tools and Strategies" in our first book called *Dyslexic AND UN-Stoppable: How Dyslexia Helps Us Create the Life of Our Dreams and How YOU Can Do It Too!*

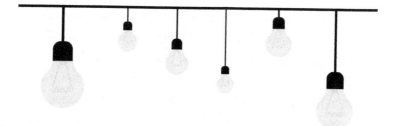

PART 2

The Yummy Recipes and Famous Quotes from Well-Known Dyslexics

Note: Some of the Well-Known Dyslexics mentioned in this cookbook have confirmed their dyslexia in the media. Others may not have been clearly identified as having dyslexia. However, researchers have reviewed available evidence, and many have come to the conclusion that they did in fact have dyslexia. We leave it to you, the reader, to decide for yourself, as our main reason for including them is to inspire children with dyslexia.

RECIPE #1

Baba's "Almost Famous" Chocolate Torpedo Sandwich

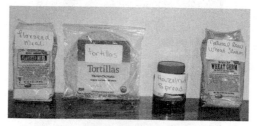

The Ingredients

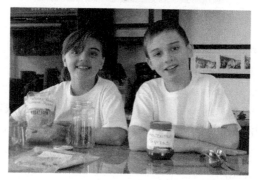

Mixing "the Crunchy Stuff"

What is "the crunchy stuff"?

Our son Félix-Alexander (FéZander) calls the wheat germ and flaxseed meal mixture "the crunchy stuff." When he was a little boy, he would say, "*Maman*, don't forget to add the crunchy stuff!"

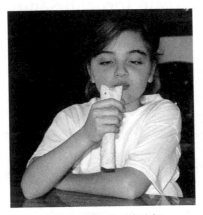

Enjoying My Sandwich!

Ingredients

1 bag of organic (whole ground) flaxseed meal

1 bag of natural raw wheat germ

1 jar of hazelnut cocoa spread (the kind with no artificial ingredients)

organic tortillas (non-GMO) or any other bread (we like spelt bread)

optional: individual packets of Amazing Grass Kidz Superfood Drink Powder (Outrageous Chocolate Flavor)

Mixing "the Crunchy Stuff"

We use recycled glass jars of wheat germ and fill them half-full with flaxseed meal and then half-full with wheat germ. Sometimes we add a few packets of Amazing Grass Kidz Superfood Drink Powder to this mixture.

Shake well until all blended.

Making the Sandwich

Spread the tortilla or bread evenly with the hazelnut cocoa spread and sprinkle 1 tablespoon of "the crunchy stuff" on top and fold the tortilla.

Enjoy immediately!

Key ingredients in this recipe:
- Flaxseed (omega-3 fatty acid, fiber)
- Wheat germ (vitamin B, fiber)
- Spelt bread (ancient healthy whole grain)
- Amazing Grass (superfood)

Visit us at www.DyslexicAndUnstoppable.com to watch the video on how to make this sandwich and to learn more about our other products.

Well-Known Dyslexic: Thomas Edison
- Inventor of the practical electric light bulb
- Inventor of the phonograph

Famous Quotes

"*I have not failed. I've just found 10,000 ways that won't work.*"

"*Our greatest weakness lies in giving up. The most certain way to succeed is always to try just one more time.*"

"*Opportunity is missed by most people because it is dressed in overalls and looks like work.*"

"*Many of life's failures are people who did not realize how close they were to success when they gave up.*"

"*Your worth consists in what you are and not in what you have.*"

"*Restlessness is discontent and discontent is the first necessity of progress. Show me a thoroughly satisfied man and I will show you a failure.*"

"*Genius is 1 percent inspiration and 99 percent perspiration.*"

To learn more about well-known dyslexics, see pictures, and much more, visit our website:

www.DyslexicAndUnstoppable.com

RECIPE #2
Tuna Melts My Way!

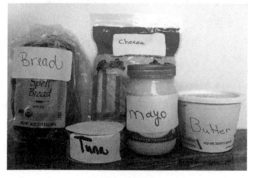

The Ingredients

Ingredients

1 can wild albacore tuna in water (no salt added)

1 tablespoon organic mayonnaise (made with free-range eggs)

½ cup cheese of your choice

4 slices of bread = 2 per person (we use organic spelt bread)

organic buttery spread

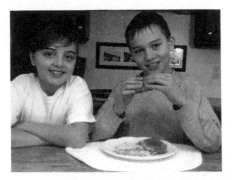

Enjoying the Tuna Melt "Cookie" Made for Me!

Making the Tuna Melt

In a big bowl, mix the following ingredients: tuna, mayonnaise, and cheese.

Spread butter on one side of each slice of bread. Place a generous portion of the tuna mixture between the bread slices, butter side out, and cook on stovetop for a few minutes on each side until golden brown.

Enjoy!

Serves 2

Key ingredients in this recipe:

- Tuna (omega-3 fatty acid, lean protein)
- Organic mayonnaise and free-range eggs (omega-3 fatty acid, choline)
- Spelt bread (ancient healthy whole grain)

Visit us at www.DyslexicAndUnstoppable.com to watch the video on how to make this tuna melt sandwich and to learn more about our other products.

Well-Known Dyslexic: Galileo Galilei

- Italian physicist
- Mathematician
- Astronomer
- Philosopher (played a major role in the Scientific Revolution)
- The father of modern observational astronomy

Famous Quotes

"*We cannot teach people anything; we can only help them discover it within themselves.*"

"*All truths are easy to understand once they are discovered; the point is to discover them.*"

"*Where the senses fail us, reason must step in.*"

"*We must say that there are as many squares as there are numbers.*"

"*Mathematics is the language in which God has written the universe.*"

"*In questions of science, the authority of a thousand is not worth the humble reasoning of a single individual.*"

To learn more about well-known dyslexics, see pictures, and much more, visit our website:

www.DyslexicAndUnstoppable.com

RECIPE #3
Super-Easy Shrimp Stir-Fry

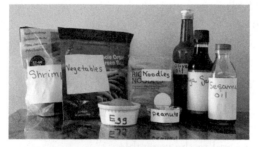

The Ingredients

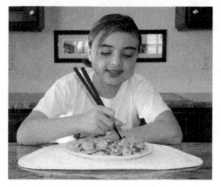

Enjoying My Stir-Fry!

Ingredients
1 bag (1 lb.) frozen uncooked wild shrimp
½ bag (1 lb.) frozen organic mixed vegetables
1 package rice noodles of your choice
4 organic free-range eggs
olive oil
pure sesame oil
organic soy sauce
peanuts

1. The Shrimp
Cook the shrimp in boiling water until pink or cooked through. Drain and return the shrimp to the covered pot to keep warm until ready to add to the vegetables.

2. The Vegetables
In the meantime, cook the frozen vegetables in 1 teaspoon of olive oil in a frying pan or wok for about 5 minutes.

3. The Noodles
Cook the noodles of your choice according to the instructions on the package.

4. The Eggs
In another small pan, cook the scrambled eggs with 1/2 teaspoon of olive oil.

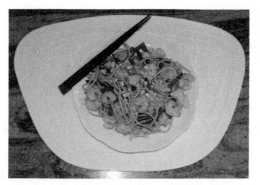

Super-Easy Shrimp Stir-Fry

When the shrimp, noodles, and eggs are all cooked perfectly, add them to the pan with the vegetables.

Add 2 teaspoons of sesame oil and soy sauce to your liking. Mix well.

Finally, sprinkle some peanuts on top.

Eat immediately!

Serves about 4.

Key ingredients in this recipe:
- Shrimp (omega-3 fatty acid, zinc, iron)
- Vegetables (fiber, vitamins and minerals)
- Egg (choline)
- Olive oil (omega-3 and omega-6 fatty acids, monounsaturated fat)
- Peanuts (essential amino acid tryptophan, vitamin B3, copper)

Visit us at www.DyslexicAndUnstoppable.com to watch the video on how to make this stir-fry and to learn more about our other products.

Well-Known Dyslexic: Benjamin Franklin

- One of the Founding Fathers of the United States
- Author
- Printer
- Politician
- Postmaster
- Scientist
- Musician
- Inventor
- Statesman
- Diplomat

Famous Quotes

"Tell me and I forget. Teach me and I remember. Involve me and I learn."

"The Constitution only gives people the right to pursue happiness. You have to catch it yourself."

"An investment in knowledge pays the best interest."

"Remember not only to say the right thing in the right place, but far more difficult still, to leave unsaid the wrong thing at the tempting moment."

"Honesty is the best policy."

"Do not fear mistakes. You will know failure. Continue to reach out."

"A penny saved is a penny earned."

To learn more about well-known dyslexics, see pictures, and much more, visit our website:

www.DyslexicAndUnstoppable.com

RECIPE #4:
Scrumptious Salmon

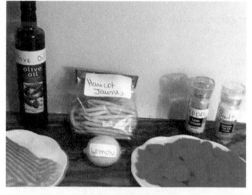

The Ingredients

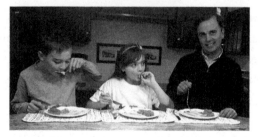

The Family Enjoying the Salmon!

Ingredients

1¼ lbs. of fresh or frozen wild salmon

1–2 lbs. organic carrots or vegetables

1 bag of organic green or yellow beans, or any vegetable of your choice

salt and pepper to taste

1 teaspoon of olive oil

juice of ½ organic lemon

1. The Salmon

Preheat the oven to 450°F.

Place the salmon in an oven-safe pan. Spread the olive oil on top of the salmon. Add salt and pepper and lemon juice to coat the fish evenly.

Bake for 15–20 minutes (depending on the thickness of your fish).

2. The Vegetables

In the meantime, steam the vegetables on the stove until tender. Alternatively, enjoy some fresh, raw vegetables.

Plate and enjoy!

Serves about 4.

Key ingredients in this recipe:
- Salmon (omega-3 fatty acid, zinc, iron)
- Vegetables (fiber, vitamins and minerals)

- Olive oil (omega-3 and omega-6 fatty acids, monounsaturated fat)
- Lemon (vitamin C, phytonutrient tangeretin)

Visit us at www.DyslexicAndUnstoppable.com to watch the video on how to make this salmon and to learn more about our other products.

Well-Known Dyslexic: Albert Einstein
- Physicist
- Discovered $E=MC^2$ (theory of relativity)

Famous Quotes

"Imagination is more important than knowledge."

"Great spirits have always encountered violent opposition from mediocre minds."

"A person who never made a mistake never tried anything new."

"Setting an example is not the main means of influencing another; it is the only means."

"Insanity: doing the same thing over and over again and expecting different results."

"If you can't explain it simply, you don't understand it well enough."

"Try not to become a man of success, but rather try to become a man of value."

To learn more about well-known dyslexics, see pictures, and much more, visit our website:

www.DyslexicAndUnstoppable.com

RECIPE #5:

An Old Favorite:
Smoked Salmon Bagel

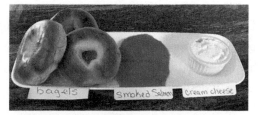

The Ingredients

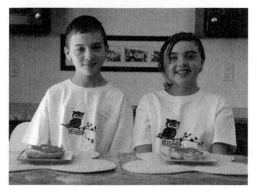

Enjoying Our Bagels!

Ingredients

bagels of your choice

1 pack wild smoked salmon

1 container organic cream cheese

1 teaspoon organic capers per person (optional)

Making the Bagels

Toast the bagels.

Spread a generous amount of cream cheese on both sides of the sliced bagel.

Add the smoked salmon on top.

Add capers, if desired.

Enjoy!

Key ingredients in this recipe:

- Salmon (omega-3 fatty acid, zinc, iron)
- Capers (fiber, antioxidants, vitamin A, niacin, riboflavin)

Visit us at www.DyslexicAndUnstoppable.com to watch the video on how to make these bagels and to learn more about our other products.

Well-Known Dyslexic: Henry Ford
- Founder of the Ford Motor Company
- A sponsor of the development of the assembly-line technique of mass production

Famous Quotes

"If you think you can do a thing or think you can't do a thing, you're right."

"Failure is simply the opportunity to begin again, this time more intelligently."

"Coming together is a beginning; keeping together is progress; working together is success."

"My best friend is the one who brings out the best in me."

"Obstacles are those frightful things you see when you take your eyes off your goal."

"Thinking is the hardest work there is, which is probably the reason why so few engage in it."

"If everyone is moving forward together, then success takes care of itself."

To learn more about well-known dyslexics, see pictures, and much more, visit our website:
www.DyslexicAndUnstoppable.com

RECIPE #6:

Meat Tacos with "Dip-Dip"

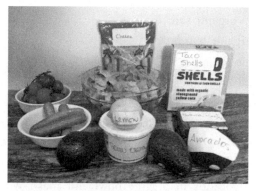

The Ingredients

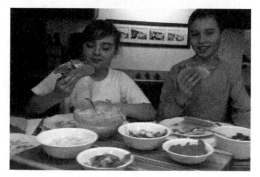

Enjoying Our Tacos!

Ingredients

1 lb. organic grass-fed ground beef (beef raised without the use
    of antibiotics or hormones)

1 box organic taco shells

2 organic avocados

1 tablespoon organic sour cream

juice of ½ organic lemon

1 cup organic tomatoes

1 cup organic cucumbers

1 head organic lettuce of your choice

½ cup shredded cheese of your choice

1. Making the "Dip-Dip"

Spoon the avocados in a large bowl and mash with a potato masher. Add the sour cream and lemon.

    Mix well!

2. The Vegetables

In the meantime, cut your tomatoes, cucumbers, and lettuce in small enough pieces so they easily fit in your taco.

3. The Meat

Cook the ground beef in a frying pan until meat is all browned (about 10 minutes on medium heat).

    While we cook the meat, we warm up the taco shells in the oven at the lowest temperature possible. On our stove, it's 170°F.

4. Assembling the Tacos

Place the meat on the bottom of the taco shell. Add the cheese, the "dip-dip," lettuce, tomatoes, and cucumbers.

Enjoy!

Serves about 4.

Key ingredients in this recipe:

- Beef (protein, iron, zinc)
- Avocados (fiber, protein, oleic acid, monounsaturated fat)
- Lemon (vitamin C, phytonutrient tangeretin)
- Tomatoes (vitamins C and A, fiber, folic acid)
- Cucumbers (fiber, vitamin K)
- Lettuce (vitamin K and A, beta-carotene)

Visit us at www.DyslexicAndUnstoppable.com to watch the video on how to make these tacos and to learn more about our other products.

Well-Known Dyslexic: Alexander Graham Bell

- Scientist
- Engineer
- Inventor of the telephone

Famous Quotes

"Sometimes we stare so long at a door that is closing that we see too late the one that is open."

"Before anything else, preparation is the key to success."

"A man, as a general rule, owes very little to what he is born with — a man is what he makes of himself."

"What this power is I cannot say; all I know is that it exists and it becomes available only when a man is in that state of mind in which he knows exactly what he wants and is fully determined not to quit until he finds it."

"God has strewn our paths with wonders and we certainly should not go through Life with our eyes shut."

To learn more about well-known dyslexics, see pictures, and much more, visit our website:

www.DyslexicAndUnstoppable.com

RECIPE #7:
Fish Tacos with "Dip-Dip"

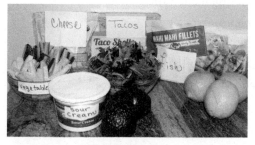

The Ingredients

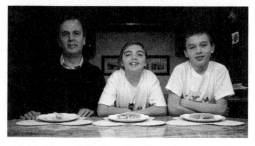

Enjoying Our Tacos!

Ingredients

1 lb. frozen wild fish (thinly sliced white fish, such as cod or
    tilapia)

1 box organic taco shells

2 organic avocados

1 tablespoon organic sour cream

juice of ½ an organic lemon

1 cup organic tomatoes

1 cup organic cucumbers

1 head organic lettuce of your choice

½ cup shredded cheese of your choice

2 organic free-range eggs, beaten

½ cup of organic enriched unbleached white flour

olive oil

1. Making the "Dip-Dip"

Spoon the avocados in a large bowl and mash with a potato masher. Add the sour cream and lemon.

Mix well!

2. Vegetables

In the meantime, cut your tomatoes, cucumbers, and lettuce in small enough pieces so they easily fit in your taco.

3. Fish

Make an assembly line:

    1 plate with the fish
    1 plate with egg mixture (uncooked)
    1 plate with ½ cup flour
    1 clean plate

Take one piece of fish at a time. Coat it with the egg mixture, and then place it in the flour, coating both sides. Place the coated fish on the clean plate and continue this process until all pieces of fish are coated. (Wash your hands afterward!)

Cook the fish in a frying pan coated with olive oil until fish is crispy on both sides (about 2 minutes per side). Next, place the fish in the oven at 350°F for 5 minutes or until cooked through.

4. The Taco Shells

While we cook the fish, we warm up the taco shells in the oven at the lowest temperature possible. On our stove, it's 170°F.

5. Assembling the Tacos

Place the fish on the bottom of the taco shell.

Add the cheese, the "dip-dip," lettuce, tomatoes, and cucumbers.

Enjoy!

Serves about 4.

Key ingredients in this recipe:

- Fish (omega-3, protein, polyunsaturated fatty acids, iodine)
- Avocados: (fiber, protein, oleic acid, monounsaturated fat)
- Lemon (vitamin C, phytonutrient tangeretin)
- Tomatoes (vitamin C and A, fiber, folic acid)
- Cucumbers (fiber, vitamin K)
- Lettuce (vitamin K and A, beta-carotene)
- Eggs (choline)
- Olive oil (omega-3 and omega-6 fatty acids, monounsaturated fat)

Visit us at www.DyslexicAndUnstoppable.com to watch the video on how to make these tacos and to learn more about our other products.

Well-Known Dyslexic: George Washington

- First president of the United States
- One of the Founding Fathers of the United States
- Commander-in-chief of the Continental Army during the American Revolutionary War

Famous Quotes

"Happiness and moral duty are inseparably connected."

"It is better to be alone than in bad company."

"Truth will ultimately prevail where there is pains to bring it to light."

"I hope I shall possess firmness and virtue enough to maintain what I consider the most enviable of all titles, the character of an honest man."

"True friendship is a plant of slow growth, and must undergo and withstand the shocks of adversity, before it is entitled to the appellation."

"My mother was the most beautiful woman I ever saw. All I am I owe to my mother. I attribute all my success in life to the moral, intellectual, and physical education I received from her."

To learn more about well-known dyslexics, see pictures, and much more, visit our website:

www.DyslexicAndUnstoppable.com

RECIPE #8:
Crêpes à la Maman

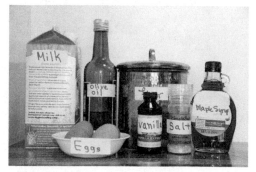

The Ingredients

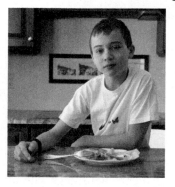 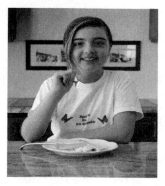

Enjoying My Crêpes!

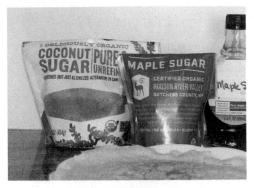

Crêpes à la Maman

Ingredients

1½ cup organic enriched unbleached white flour

3 cups organic fat-free milk

4 organic free-range eggs

2 teaspoons olive oil (plus more for cooking)

a pinch of Himalayan salt

2 teaspoons pure vanilla

organic maple syrup, organic pure maple sugar, or organic
    coconut sugar

organic buttery spread

Making the Batter

In a big bowl, mix the following ingredients: flour, eggs, salt, olive
oil, and vanilla.

To this batter, add ONLY 1 cup of milk, and mix until all
the ingredients are blended well without any lumps. When the

mixture is all smooth, add the remaining milk and place the batter in the fridge for 30 minutes.

Thirty minutes later, bring the batter out of the fridge and mix well, as some of the batter may have settled on the bottom of the bowl during refrigeration.

Heat a large frying pan, crêpe pan, or hot plate on medium-high. Add 1 teaspoon of olive oil and about ⅓ cup of batter (about ¾ of a ladle) into heated pan.

Spread the mixture as thinly as possible. (Remember, these are French crêpes, not pancakes. The thinner the better for this recipe.)

Cook for a few minutes on each side.

Repeat the process until the batter is all used.

You may find that you need to coat the pan with olive oil periodically as you make your crêpes (to prevent sticking).

In the meantime, keep the crêpes warm in the oven at the lowest temperature possible.

We top these crêpes with any of the following:

- Maple syrup
- A dollop of butter and maple sugar
- A dollop of butter and coconut sugar

Enjoy!

Serves about 4 (about 15 crêpes in total).

Key ingredients in this recipe:
- Olive oil (omega-3 and omega-6 fatty acids, monounsaturated fat)
- Eggs (choline)
- Milk (protein, phosphorus, riboflavin, niacin)
- Vanilla (antioxidants)

Visit us at www.DyslexicAndUnstoppable.com to watch the video on how to make these crêpes and to learn more about our other products.

Well-Known Dyslexic: Leonardo da Vinci
- "Renaissance Man"
- Painter
- Sculptor
- Architect
- Musician
- Mathematician
- Engineer
- Inventor
- Anatomist
- Geologist
- Cartographer

- Botanist
- Writer

Famous Quotes

"Simplicity is the ultimate sophistication."

"I love those who can smile in trouble, who can gather strength from distress, and grow brave by reflection. 'Tis the business of little minds to shrink, but they whose heart is firm, and whose conscience approves their conduct, will pursue their principles unto death."

"There are three classes of people: those who see, those who see when they are shown, and those who do not see."

"Water is the driving force of all nature."

"Where the spirit does not work with the hand, there is no art."

"Why does the eye see a thing more clearly in dreams than the imagination when awake?"

To learn more about well-known dyslexics, see pictures, and much more, visit our website:

www.DyslexicAndUnstoppable.com

RECIPE #9:
Super-Easy Banana Bread

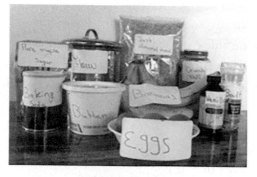

The Ingredients

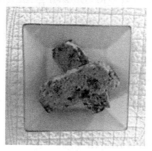

Super-Easy Banana Bread

Ingredients
4 ripe smashed bananas
⅓ cup melted organic buttery spread
½ cup organic pure maple sugar
1 organic free-range egg, beaten
1 teaspoon pure vanilla
1 teaspoon baking soda
a pinch of Himalayan salt
1½ cups of organic enriched unbleached white flour
1 tablespoon Just Almond Meal
1 teaspoon of "the Crunchy Stuff" (see recipe #1 for details)
olive oil (to coat the pan)

Making the Bread
Preheat the oven to 350°F.

In a large bowl, add the following ingredients: bananas, the buttery spread, sugar, egg, vanilla, baking soda, flour, salt, Just Almond Meal, and "the Crunchy Stuff." Mix with a wooden spoon, then pour the mixture into a loaf pan coated with olive oil.

Bake for 45 minutes. Enjoy!

Makes one loaf.

Key ingredients in this recipe:
- Banana (fiber, tryptophan)
- Eggs (choline)
- Vanilla (antioxidants)

- Olive oil (omega-3 and omega-6 fatty acids, monounsaturated fat)
- Flaxseeds (omega-3 fatty acid, fiber)
- Wheat germ (vitamin B, fiber)

Visit us at www.DyslexicAndUnstoppable.com to watch the video on how to make this banana bread and to learn more about our other products.

Well-Known Dyslexic: Pablo Picasso

One of the greatest and most influential artists of the twentieth century

- Co-founder of Cubism, the avant-garde art movement

Famous Quotes

"*Only put off until tomorrow what you are willing to die having left undone.*"

"*All children are artists. The problem is how to remain an artist once he grows up.*"

"*Action is the foundational key to all success.*"

"*Some painters transform the sun into a yellow spot, others transform a yellow spot into the sun.*"

"*Painting is a blind man's profession. He paints not what he sees, but what he feels, what he tells himself about what he has seen.*"

"Everything you can imagine is real."
"To draw you must close your eyes and sing."
"It takes a long time to become young."

To learn more about well-known dyslexics, see pictures, and much more, visit our website:

www.DyslexicAndUnstoppable.com

RECIPE #10:

Chloé's "Surprise" Peanut Butter Cookies

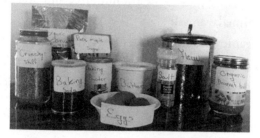

The Ingredients

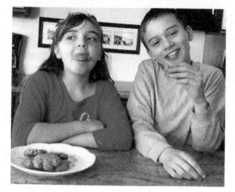

Enjoying Our Cookies!

Ingredients

½ cup melted organic buttery spread

¼ cup organic pure maple sugar

½ cup organic coconut sugar

1 organic free-range egg, beaten

¾ teaspoon baking soda

½ teaspoon baking powder (aluminum free and double acting)

a pinch of Himalayan salt

1¼ cups organic enriched unbleached white flour

½ cup organic peanut butter (non-GMO)

1 teaspoon of "the Crunchy Stuff" (see recipe #1 for details)

Making the Cookies

Preheat the oven to 350°F.

In a large bowl, add the following ingredients: maple and coconut sugars, buttery spread, peanut butter, egg, baking soda, baking powder, flour, salt, and "the Crunchy Stuff."

Mix with a wooden spoon until well blended.

Place the mixture in the fridge for 10 minutes before cooking.

Form little balls with the dough. Place the balls on your cookie sheet covered with parchment paper. With a fork, press on the balls to flatten them in a crisscross pattern. Bake for 8–10 minutes.

Enjoy!

Makes about 10–15 cookies.

Key ingredients in this recipe:

- Eggs (choline)
- Olive oil (omega-3 and omega-6 fatty acids, monounsaturated fat)
- Flaxseeds (omega-3 fatty acid, fiber)
- Wheat germ (vitamin B, fiber)
- Maple sugar (mega-antioxidant, anti-inflammatory)
- Coconut sugar (antioxidants, and the following phytonutrients: polyphenols, flavonoids, and anthocyanidin)
- Peanut butter (antioxidants, tryptophan, fiber)

Visit us at www.DyslexicAndUnstoppable.com to watch the video on how to make these cookies and to learn more about our other products.

Epilogue

The fact that you are interested in this book probably means that you are questioning whether you or someone you love has dyslexia. Having a clear picture of what dyslexia looks like and knowing the signs and symptoms will help us connect the dots and identify dyslexia sooner, which in return gives our dyslexic children a greater chance of successfully overcoming it.

Every dyslexic is different, but here are some of the difficulties commonly associated with dyslexia:

- Reading aloud
- Decoding words
- Learning spelling words
- Memorizing basic math facts and timed tests
- Laborious handwriting
- Mixing uppercase and lowercase letters when writing
- Remembering the alphabet
- Speech issues
- Fidgetiness

- Fine motor skills
- Learning to tell time

Another aspect of dyslexia is called *dysgraphia*. Dysgraphia simply means the impairment of the ability to write. Following are some of the symptoms of dysgraphia. Not every dyslexic has dysgraphia. (Our son has dysgraphia, so that is why we included these signs in this book.)

- Difficulty gripping a pencil comfortably while writing
- Unusual wrist, body, and paper orientations
- Excessive erasures
- Mixed uppercase and lowercase letters
- Inconsistent form and size of letters, or unfinished letters
- Misuse of lines and margins
- Inefficient speed of copying
- Inattentiveness over details when writing
- Poor handwriting legibility
- Handwriting abilities that may interfere with spelling and written composition
- Difficulty translating ideas to writing, sometimes using the wrong words altogether
- Difficulty spelling words correctly and consistently
- Difficulty aligning numbers correctly while doing math problems

- Difficulty using silverware properly
- Difficulty with buttons and zippers
- Difficulty tying shoes
- Laborious writing and copying
- Difficulty doing two tasks at once (such as thinking and writing at the same time)

Learning the signs of dyslexia early will help parents be better advocates for their children. Making the connection between their children's struggles and the services needed is the first step to overcoming dyslexia.

We want to remind you, as parents, how lucky you are to have a dyslexic child. Dyslexic children are gifts. Keep empowering your child and see him or her become UN-Stoppable.

After years of taking self-development courses, the one thing we learned to really appreciate is the gift of HEALTH! You can have all the money in the world, all the material things you desire, a closet full of shoes, the "right" toys, and the "right" cars—BUT if you don't have your health, you don't have anything!

Taking the time out of your busy life to make good food choices is crucial if you want to enjoy a long and healthy life and keep your brain working properly.

Our hope is that this book inspires you to enjoy a healthy lifestyle and healthy eating habits. Choosing to make healthier choices is the key to success.

Check out the foods you eat and read those ingredient lists. Get informed! Is it always easy to make changes? Of course not! Is it necessary? You be the judge!

One step at a time, we can do anything we put our minds to!

Health is by far the biggest gift we were given. Take good care of it. You'll be glad you did!

Now that you have a better understanding of why we chose these recipes and nutrients to maximize our son's ability to overcome dyslexia, it's your turn to take these simple and nutritious ingredients to create yummy recipes that your dyslexic child (and family) will enjoy. Send us your creations, and we will add them to our website so other parents can try them out (www. DyslexicAndUnstoppable.com).

Acknowledgments

You know the traditional African proverb: "It takes a village to raise a child." Well, it also takes a village to spread a message, and write and publish books. We have so many people to thank. First, we want to thank Morgan James Publishing for believing in us and being willing to see the world through a dyslexic's point of view. "As dyslexics, we love visuals" is Lucie's motto. The more bolds, highlights, pictures, and textboxes we can add, the BETTER!

Big thanks also to Amanda Rooker, our editor at SplitSeed, for understanding and working with our vision for our books. It is such a pleasure and delight to collaborate with people who get our mission at Dyslexic AND UN-Stoppable.

Last but not least, thanks to our two awesome kids, Cookie and FéZander, and our families for their constant love and support. You all rock!

This journey to empower dyslexic children to become UN-Stoppable has put some truly amazing people in our path, and we are forever grateful to have met them all. Wow, what a ride! And this is just the beginning . . .

About the Authors

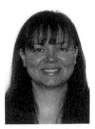

Lucie M. Curtiss, RN, is a dyslexic and the co-founder of Dyslexic AND UN-Stoppable and co-author of the *Dyslexic AND UN-Stoppable* book series. She's also a mother, pediatric nurse, entrepreneur, and business manager of a thriving pediatric practice. For the past decade she's successfully helped her son overcome dyslexia. Her mission is to empower dyslexic children to become UN-Stoppable and overcome dyslexia by rediscovering their inner power and realizing they are SMART.

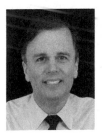

Douglas C. Curtiss, MD, FAAP, is a board-certified, Yale-trained pediatrician with over 18 years of experience. He has helped thousands of parents navigate the school system and advocate for their dyslexic children. He is the co-founder of Dyslexic AND UN-Stoppable and co-author of the

Dyslexic AND UN-Stoppable book series. He was trained in traditional Western medicine, and as an avid student of personal development, he began to look at complementary medicine techniques to incorporate into his practice. When his son was discovered to be dyslexic, Dr. Curtiss worked with his wife, Lucie Curtiss, to find the best methods, both traditional and complementary, to help their son overcome dyslexia. After seeing the results firsthand of his son's success, Doug has teamed up with his wife to help parents of kids with dyslexia find the tools and strategies and make educated choices to help their children rise to their fullest potential.

To Learn More

To learn more about Lucie M. Curtiss and Dr. Douglas Curtiss, and to watch our videos and leave comments, visit www. DyslexicAndUnStoppable.com.

Like our page on Facebook: www.facebook.com/ DyslexicUnStoppable.

Subscribe to our YouTube channel: www.youtube.com/user/ DyslexicUnstoppable.

Follow us on Twitter: @curtissdc

Please leave feedback where you bought the book. Thank you!

References

http://www.rottentomatoes.com/celebrity/albert_einstein/
    pictures/
http://www.brainyquote.com/quotes/authors/a/albert_einstein.
    html
http://www.bolderlifefestival.com/wp-content/uploads/2013/02/
    Thomas-Edison.png
http://www.usmilitaryhalloffame.org/Members/Individual/
    GeorgeWashington.aspx
http://www.pinterest.com/pin/474496510711241908/
http://en.wikipedia.org/wiki/Leonardo_da_Vinci
https://www.google.com
http://www.ask.com/question/what-is-henry-ford-famous-for
http://www.biography.com/people/pablo-picasso-9440021
http://www.ask.com/question/what-is-galileo-galilei-famous-for
http://www.quotationspage.com/quote/40028.html
https://www.goodreads.com/author/quotes/14190.Galileo_
    Galilei

http://www.guruhabits.com/wp/wp-content/uploads/2012/10/
    john-lennon-imagine.jpg
http://www.thelancet.com/journals/lancet/article/
    PIIS0140673607613063/abstract
http://www.ncbi.nlm.nih.gov/pmc/articles/PMC1029619
http://www.dyslexic.org.uk/research-nutrition.html
http://www.ncbi.nlm.nih.gov/pubmed/24381967
http://www.ncbi.nlm.nih.gov/pubmed/9368235

CPSIA information can be obtained at www.ICGtesting.com
Printed in the USA
BVOW11s1536130915

417694BV00004B/7/P